ME AND MY
BARBER

The Successful Barbers' Strategies

By

Franklin Ndubuisi Ahaotu

i

CONTENTS

PREFACE

What's the nature of your Barbershop? Are you aware that Barbers are caregivers? This book will practically teach you how you can succeed in Barbershop Business.

A few moral obligations that define a good barber, Clipper maintenance, and many ways a barber can make money have been carefully examined; with specific emphasis on Barbering career-related issues that a barber should Know before establishing a Barbershop.

The author has articulated excellently, his personal experience to help Barbers and barbershop hopefuls in their journey to success.

You too "...can make the barbershop a place to gather business wisdom"

"You have to be very observant in handling different types of hairs as no two individual's hair grows the same way. Some have extra hair in the ear region, others a little below the neck; some at the fore, while the rest may have theirs, a little above the eyebrows, etc. Always check for these hidden spots that elude inexperience Barbers, as you render your services. Confirm that no hair is left where they're not needed."

CHAPTER 1

Nature Of Barbershop Services

The word Barber is derived from a Latin word meaning "beard." A Barber in this write up would mean anyone, who is in the business of cutting hairs. Barbershop, therefore, is operating such a business, especially for men and boys.

The primary reason for opening a Barbershop is to have a place where people will come to have their hairs cut and styled, shaved, or trimmed. But today, most Barbershops offer other services.

Apart from providing a haircut, dying and styling of hairs can as well be done inside a Barbershop; for men and sometimes for both men and women. So, if you're a barber, you'll focus on carrying out grooming services especially for men with a few exceptions, while that of a Hairstylist involves both males and females. It does mean that both barbers and stylists can cut, color, curl, or style hair. Only barbers, though, majors in razor shaves for men.

As preliminary advice to prepare you for this great job, I want to let you know that the art of Barbering is not an easy job.

Unlike what you had thought before now, haircutting is a nerve-racking act that requires a lot of concentration. Very few occupations are as tricky as this, simply because you're having constant personal interactive contact with different individuals whose opinion is as important as your income.

Barbers are not like fashion designers. For instance, a fashion designer only works on fabric to achieve customers' needs, and as such an amateur designer can take a difficult job to a more experienced colleague for sewing and still gets credit for the job since the customer might not know exactly who does the-sewing.

A barber does not have such a luxury, as his job requires an on-the-spot assessment. And so, in case you're having a little difficulty blending well on this job, in terms of your skill level, do not be discouraged as almost all who are today mentors in Barbering was once in your shoe.

If you've decided to run a Barbershop, it's a great business I must say. Having acquired the right skill and must have worked in a Barbershop for some time, you think you're good at it; and you want to start operating your shop. One of the first things to consider is how you will operate the business.

Are you going to hire a barber or barbers, at this point, or just run the shop alone-at least for the main time? The answer to this question is largely dependent on the size, or rather the scale of your business; and what you want to achieve as part of your business goal.

Many factors will work together to determine how the shop will operate when you finally start operation. Some of these factors are what we'll discuss here.

Running a Small Barbershop:-

I assume you've decided to set up a small Barbershop that will have one or more barbers. Assuming also that you have concluded that you're going to manage this great business, which I strongly recommend; you have to develop a passion for the job. This passion will keep you going when you begin to attend to first-time customers, who are usually antagonistic.

That is where your first impression will come in handy. As a rule, I'd advise you to fix your price base on the prevailing price within the locality, despite how good you think your services are; but then, it should be reviewed if need be, as you develop your customer base.

The reason is that if you charge a fee that is too high, only those who can afford the bill will patronize your Barbershop; and it's very difficult to know if this number will be enough to sustain the business.

It's usually a bad idea to set a high price at the beginning; only to reduce it shortly after. Let's say $15, and after four months of operation, you reduce it to $12.

A sudden price reduction like this will suggest inconsistency; and is usually interpreted by customers, as lacking in focus and unprofessionalism.

One salient area that you must not compromise is the working condition of your equipment. Your clipper should be sharp and friendly on the skin, usually achieved when it's properly aligned and oiled before use. Sharp but unaligned clippers can be very harsh on the skin and as such should be avoided.

If you operate in a place that usually has an irregular supply of electricity, then be sure to keep, on standby, a private power generator that is in good condition.

Thank God your Barbershop is now running, you're always on-ground to attend to customers, and a good number of persons seem to have approved your services; now it appears as if you may not be able to take on the increasing number of customers, or that you're simply feeling stressed up; being that you come to the shop early and close late. So you need another Barber to support you.

Let me now advise you on the fact that no matter how good you think such a person is, as you're thinking to hire him or her, never rely on that person, in terms of management; especially, if he or she is not part of the ownership structure in a way. The logic here is that unless such a person has something to lose financially if the business goes under, he or she may not be as serious as you would want.

This is because, most of them take this occupation as a transit kind of a job, and are never serious with the business until they upgrade from just being a regular freelance Barber to a Barbershop owner.

This advice is necessary because, from my years of experience in the industry, I've observed that most of the barbers that I've employed, on this freelance kind of engagement, are not always committed to growing the business; rather are just concern with making money and building a personal relationship with their customers; and as such prefers to work on freelance bases.

That is why most times when they move away from your Barbershop, their loyal customers move with them.

Let your relationship with them be clearly defined though. Thus, are you going to pay them for their services or allow them to remit a particular percentage of their income to you?

Neither of them is bad anyway, based on its advantages and disadvantages; but I'd suggest you allow them to remit a percentage to you for a start until you can trust them enough to include them in your management team.

Freelance Barbers can as well run your Barbershop down with their attitude to customers: if you're not very observant. So be sure to caution them, if possible remove any barber that does not give a damn about how a customer feels about his hair.

But if you're planning a bigger Barbershop that would start up with at least three barbers, then you should set up a good management team with a proper accounting system.

A receptionist/cashier and a cleaner should come in handy, with proper ticketing of customers. Remember that if you're running a small Barbershop, you may decide to be the cleaner and cashier/receptionist, regardless of whether you have freelance Barbers, working with you or not.

Location:-Where you open your Barbershop is very important and would determine the success or failure of the business.

The best place to open a Barbershop is within a residential area, against the commercial environment. Opening a Barbershop in a commercial area means that your target customers will be mainly those in transit and most shops in such locations usually combine Barbershops with another kind of business. E.g Barbershop and studio services

Similarly, a Barbershop located along a highway with a traffic speed limit of between

60k/h and above is not ideal, as the shop will mostly be noticed by those walking on foot, because of the speed at which vehicles drive by; thereby limiting the number of persons who will see your signpost.

Your Barbershop will be fine if you're situated on a densely populated street, with slow-moving traffic; a busy junction preferable. If it's possible, avoid the unnecessary competition that usually arises when you locate your shop at a proximity that is within 100metres between you and already existing Barbershop.

How you arrange the Barbershop is simply your choice but it should reflect the trend and class of people within the locality.

Let me also add that because you're expected to open early and close late, it's also advisable that you operate your Barbershop closer to your home.

The reason is that despite your busy schedule, sooner you'll receive a call at an odd hour, from a loyal customer who will request for your service, either earlier before time or later, when you're almost done with the day's business.

One fast way of losing such people is to let them know that you're angry with them, over the call. So while you may not satisfy all of them that will call at an odd hour, still find time to apologize for your inability.

CHAPTER 2

Barbers are Caregivers

I've heard a lot of people say that Barbers are not just haircut experts. As they provide a kind of psychological relaxation to individual customers, interact with them in a way that helps the relaxation process.

This presupposes that their usual easygoing personality is something anyone who wants to succeed in the profession must imbibe.

As it has been widely observed that their success does not only depend on their haircutting skills but on the kind of environment they create for their customers

Now as a strategy you may decide to welcome every client with a good morning, good afternoon, or good evening as the case may be, as they walk into the shop. But then the real challenge is when you're busy with a customer, and other customers are coming in. Though naturally, whoever comes in has to wait. You have to go beyond greeting to talk to them politely.

It would be more rewarding if you have a respectable sense of humor: an honest joke will make customers view you and your shop as a fun place to hang out while waiting for a haircut.

Entertainment:- There are many ways you can entertain your customers; this includes those on standby, and the ones already receiving a haircut. A television set, a good sound system, or a newspaper/magazine is the three major ways you can set the ball rolling.

Some folks may decide to invest in all these three; this is good, especially if you can regulate how you use it; so that it does not create a nuisance, rather than relaxation that it was meant to achieve. You can do this by projecting one, at a time.

Again, the type of entertainment you'd concentrate on would be determined by some factors, which include the nature of your potential customers, your location, trends within the locality, etc.

For instance, if you're located within a school environment, where a lot of young people wouldn't mind walking into your barbershop, regardless of whether they're having a haircut or not; then you have to regulate your **TV** set; otherwise you will be contending with many who will naturally occupy your limited seats when they'd glue their eyes on your TV set; including those who are your customers, but do not have any business being in the shop at such a time.

Handling this set of people is sometimes a serious dilemma for the Barbershop operator, who may not necessarily want to embarrass such a category of persons; even as their TV viewing attitude seriously constitutes a nuisance for him or her.

To curtail their activities, I recommend that you keep the TV set off at a certain period, and only switch on if customers present, so demanded.

Your sound system should be in good condition; some customers may want the volume high while others would prefer a low sound output. The right word here would be moderation.

Let me also add that you should psychologically observe individual customer's emotions at every point in time. This's intuitively determined by their age bracket and interest.

Elderly/educated customers will find your current newspapers interesting; just as sports enthusiasts will, on sports magazines.

Personally inspire conversation, if you feel that the environment is boring, by doing the following: changing the TV set channel, to suit the category of persons present; discussing a particular news headline, or still, cautiously following the lyric of a song in a modest way that would entertain customers.

These things are done unconsciously by most barbers, because of their passion for the job.

Clean Barbershop and Cleaning:-An uninteresting fact about some barbershop owners is the fact that they don't have a good clean-up culture. Rather than opening a beautiful barbershop and watch it go rusty, while not start moderately and keep upgrading till you set a reasonable standard. You need not be told that hairs must be swept off after each barbing section; or once you're in the clear of customers.

All your tools, including clippers, scissors, hairbrushes, combs, etc. should be regularly cleaned and sterilized.

Though health-conscious customers would still want you to do an on-the-spot cleaning of these tools, before using it on them, it's ethically and hygienically good to do the cleaning in advance. This, apart from keeping the environment free of bacteria, will instill confidence in your customers.

Human hairs on the floor usually appear messy most times, so be sure to sweep off the floor at all times: as soon as you have the opportunity to do so.

In fact, as a barber that wants to progress in this profession and make a reasonable profit from it; you're required to adhere to the basic legal standard for cleanliness; just like other cosmetologists.

Though these legal guidelines may be way out of your real cost in terms of budgeting, it would not only help you in avoiding legal issues in the future but would give your barbershop a good representation in the minds of your customers.

Proper arrangements of Props with the doors open or close as the case may be, to ensure an airy atmosphere. Your air conditioner, fan, etc. should be in good condition; using disinfectant regularly, to achieve a decent and clean environment.

Then there's this aspect of the cleanliness that would mess up your barbershop unless you're aware of it. For the sake of nomenclature, I will call it the "Body odor syndrome".

I guess you don't need to be told that you're constantly in close contact with different individuals that have their different taste and preferences. If you're a **chain-smoker**, for instance, you have to be sure that you don't inconvenience your customers with tobacco smell.

Though no scene Barbershop owner would want you to take up a client if you're taking a drug, excessive alcoholic drinking habit can also give you an unpleasant smell that may irritate others.

It might not be anything but outright poor personal hygiene habit that is given you off anytime you're in contact with your customer. That's why you need to be aware of all these so that your smartness and creativity will work together with your skill to give the desired result.

Have also a specified business hour:- Do not forget to let your customers know your business hour so that you don't get a call from a customer when you're still in bed; or when you're done for the day.

And again, it's simple to advertise a particular business hour or operation timetable, the real deal is sticking to your schedule. If you fail regularly to observe the already advertised schedule, you will be subtly killing the business; as you'll be disappointing many, who will quickly interpret it as not being serious with the business

Also, having a clear business hour and sticking to it will help your customers plan their haircut time. Let me also add that not being at your duty post (the Barbershop) regularly is a bad way to run a Barbershop.

Add More Value with Extra services:- You have to be very observant in handling different types of hairs, as no two individual's hair grows the same way. Some have extra hair in the ear region, others a little below the neck; some at the fore, or even a little above the eyebrows, etc. Always check for these hidden spots that elude inexperience Barbers, as you render your services. Confirm that no hair is left where it's not needed.

As a rule, and a tested fact, be satisfied with the job that you've done on him or her before you let that customer out of his seat; and never depend on the customer's opinion, or asked for his final approval.

It does not speak well of the Barber's creative decision; especially when himself (the Barber) is satisfied with the output.

An exception to this is, if you observe psychologically, that your customer is not satisfied. In such instances, your aim of asking his opinion would be to correct an already formed bad impression, with a subtle promise to make up for your mistake in the future.

While trimming hair on certain hidden spots, your soft touches, subtle smiles, and cheerful disposition create a positive impression that is like extra services that will keep the customer coming back.

Apart from how you handle the hairs, you should always find a way of providing something that will delight your customer; because his chance of returning next time is very high. That is why as a professional barber, you should understand the concept of hair cutting and have a special skill, peculiar to you alone.

Attend to Needs of Non-Customers:- This category of persons includes but not limited to women (if it's not a Unisex shop) who do not have any reason to cut hair, but sometimes find their way into the shop; either accompanying a customer or just there to apply powder, use your mirror or some other reasons. This group of persons though may be distracting, or simply annoying.

Annoying? Yes! They can also be useful to you: In most cases, they may be helpful in word-of-mouth promotion; and sometimes even refer people to your shop if they're ok with how you treat them.

Agreed, it's more often difficult to satisfy this faceless group of persons who do not add to the financial growth of the business. You should just make every effort to respect their demand for free service, even as most of them make it a habit, thereby constituting a nuisance.

Just take solace in the fact that they may give a good review of your Barbershop that would get you a more loyal customer.

Your barbershop should be well lighted:-

By now you must have known the advantages of the proper use of lighting in your shop; both for proper visibility and customer's comfort. Apart from the beautiful scenery that lighting creates, you will always need a very bright light while cutting hairs, even in the daytime. So your light should be as bright as possible. A traditional Barbershop in my locality usually designs their shop with white wall paints because of the reflective nature of white light on a white background.

But with the advent of the modern lighting system, many barbershop designers have deviated from that norm to something very colorful, especially with the recent progress in an interior decorating industry that saw the production of very beautiful wallpapers and wallpaper tiles that are being used today, in place of wall painting.

CHAPTER 3

Succeeding In Barbershop

Operating a lucrative barbershop depends on some factors, including your skill, your location, owner's business insight, consistency, work ethics, etc.

Knowing how to creatively give a customer a nice appearance is just one aspect, though very important; Skill would help you get hold of customers. However, your aim should be to make them loyal customers through sound customer relations.

> *"You can make the barbershop a place to gather business wisdom...,"*

a mentor once suggested.

Earlier, I talked about discussing with your customers. Are you sure you can strike a good conversation if you don't have anything useful and interesting to discuss? If there is any strategy that I employed perfectly in the success of my Barbershop, this one I'm about to reveal should be the first and most exciting tactic that I used:

Emotionally connect with your customers:- Allowing your customers to be emotionally connected to your personal life, motivations, dreams, and aspirations; as a Barbershop business strategy, is probably a tactical and salient area that goes unnoticed in the sub-consciousness of customers.

Whether you believe it or not, there is always an emotional reason (apart from physical benefit or skill,) why someone would prefer to have you as his Barber, rather than another person.

More often, I've heard folks say things like "I like him because he is hardworking," "I like him because he is a nice person," and "I like him because he is always happy and not easily offended" etc. Some would frankly tell you that they don't know why they like that Barber.

These are comments you would hear from Barbershop customers that are emotionally connected with their Barbers.

Now, how you get them to be emotionally involved with you, would depend on how you use your skills in unfolding that historical aspect of your personal life that would attract sympathy, trust, jealousy, confidence, etc. of your customers; thereby winning them individually, as friends.

And each of them would always see you as a personal friend since you've shared an aspect of your positive secret with them. I will tell you a story of how I was able to get emotionally connected with many of my customers.

After completing my higher education, with upper credit in Mass communication, I was physically and mentally prepared to join the workforce, and pursue my journalism career.

But four months of intensive job hunt to no avail was enough to sign of despair that made me look the way of entrepreneurship. My best option then was a Barbershop, which I did with great hope; having worked as a freelance Barber for up to five years, while pursuing my journalism career.

Again, before then, I had written two novels, which I had to place in a strategic position in my shop, where everyone who entered the shop could see them.

Unlike what you may be thinking, I don't have to tell each of them my story as they walk in; rather, I'd subtly advertised myself around the shop, in a way that elevated my status beyond my Barbershop.

From time to time, I'd find myself answering customer's questions from my Novels. Some would want to know when I learned the art of barbering and why I prefer it, despite having a sound academic background.

The gory tells of unemployment in my country was enough reason for my customers to sympathize with me, and as such, was ready to make me grow in my vision of adding value to society by creating a positive impact, rather than going into crime like other misinformed youths.

In this instance, my achievement as a qualified but unemployed journalist, and again a published novelist, created friends for me; some of who either saw me as a role model or as someone worthy of being an associate.

At a point, I got tired of hearing encouraging words like "I like your courage, keep it up to my friend" etc. By this, my charisma was indirectly marketing my business and even helping in making my Barbering skills more attractive and acceptable by them.

Understand customer's hairstyle:- if you want to succeed in this, make sure you understand a customer's hairstyle instruction before you start clipping off the hairs. There are names for different styles.

These, you have to learn and understand, to avoid misunderstanding. Let me also add that most persons would quote a particular style, not knowing exactly what the style looks like or not knowing how they would appear on the style that they have asked you to do on them.

The creative approach to this is to, where necessary, cut off a section of hairs and ask a customer to approve before you proceed, just to be sure both of you are on the same page. If possible also, as you manipulate the hair, equally ask for an opinion to see if you're following the instructions; especially if it's a first-time customer.

Are all these necessary? Someone would ask. Yes, it's simply because, at each stage in the delivery process, your customer's opinion is important. All you need to learn is how to ask the right question, most reasonably.

Show genuine interest in issues concerning your customers, to build a relationship that will encourage them to return.

Always appear friendly, and where necessary express sympathy with their problems.

As regards interaction, though you must know your environment: the nature and composition of those who patronize you, and know what issue to avoid discussing. If you're in a very religious neighborhood, you should try to flow along with the prevailing mood rather than frivolous gist that may disconnect you from them. That is why it's essential to know your customers well.

Avoid Using Painful Clipper:- human skin is very sensitive to a sharp object, this includes the head region. That is why I teach young learner barbers to handle human hair the way they would handle a fresh egg.

While cutting hairs, some of your customers would complain of your blade being too painful and would demand that it be readjusted; while some would simply endure it, and may never come back to your shop; simply because they were not comfortable with your instrument.

Avoid this scenario by making sure that your blades are well sharpened and correctly aligned before you begin with a customer. If you must use a clipper that you think is a little rough on the skin, you should be very careful and very observant of the person's reaction to it.

Control your temperament:-Yes! As a human, the tendency to react negatively to a perceived or actual threat to one's peace is an issue, especially if you think that whoever is doing so is trying to ridicule you; or that it's been done on purpose that may not be obvious to an observer.

Now I will tell you a little story of what usually transpires between Barbers and some of their customers.

Yes, you've just resumed the weekend's services that are usually hectic, because of the volume of persons that normally cut their hairs within this period. You're through with the first customer, three persons were already seated on the waiting chair, and then this young fellow with a sophisticated hairstyle takes his turn and seats on the Barber's chair.

His face isn't familiar; it's probably his first time in your shop.

Despite asking the initial question of direction before kick-starting the cutting process, with just a few clips on his hair, you notice that this customer is not comfortable; either because of his facial expression or just his body posture. To make matters worst, he seems to be turning awkwardly on a regular interval, thereby making the hair styling process, a little cumbersome.

On two occasions you had to pause and ask if there is anything you are not doing right. He responded that you should continue.

Being that two more people are intently waiting for you and his uncomfortable disposition is, unfortunately, prolonging his time on the seat, you decide to ignore his uncanny behavior, and continue on your planned design for his hair. Halfway down the line, he explodes embarrassingly.

"What's this?" he said, referring to what you're doing on his hair. At this juncture, you're speechless, angry, and disappointed. Still, in a state of bewilderment, you decide to ask what the problem was.

Now, depending on his level of respect for you, you'd probably get a yell of disapproval or subtle but embarrassing words, which often come in the following statement: "You've spoiled the hair."

And as the saying goes, "customers are always right!" you start thinking. This scenario if not well handled could make you lose the said customer in the future, and even those already waiting for their turn on your seat; especially if they're also first-timers.

It probably wasn't your fault that this man's hairstyle was not accurately done; it may have occurred simply because this fellow did not believe that you could do it right, and as such made it even more difficult for you to add more creativity in what you were doing.

This is where your temperament control comes to play. The hard-won lesson here is that while you cannot stop entirely a situation like this from occurring, at least, you could learn to accept and acknowledge the person's opinion in a manner that will make you win him or her over as a friend; not as a customer now.

You never know, perhaps by just being a friend, he may want to give you a second chance in the future.

On many occasions as a professional Barber, I've turned this kind of customers into loyal customers, thereafter. That's the magic that only a few professional Barbers know. Though several others may know this as well, more often, would not be able to apply the trick, due to their low tolerance to this issue of temperament.

The very moment barbers dread most is when a customer has to return to their Barbershop to complain of a very poor haircut. In most cases, these unsatisfied customers would want their hair re-done by another Barber in the same shop, or another barbershop if it's only you in your shop. It's quite a humiliating moment for almost all Barbers.

So do well to avoid this kind of scenario. Though once in a while you may have a case of an unsatisfied customer, but when it becomes frequent, you should know that you need to work on your skill.

Be skillful and Smart Barber:-one of the things that barbershop owners and your customers as well, would use to access your skill level is the speed at which you can handle a client's hair. Let me also remind you that while many persons would prefer that you take it slowly because of the pleasurable effect of just sitting and have somebody twiddle on your hair, this slow approach does not always help you in your earning.

Recalling my active years as a barber, I still remember how some persons would literary tell you not to rush their hairstyle. They're suggesting that you spend the whole day on their hair, but are telling you to be creative while handling their hair. By this, I'm saying that the end should justify the means.

Barbershop owners also prefer fast and efficient Barbers. Indeed you need to be a smart Barber because it will reduce the duration a customer will spend in your Barbershop and as well, increase your income, as you would be attending to more customers than a slow Barber.

Naturally, the speed at which you finish perfectly a hairstyle, creates a good impression about your barbing skill, even to those yet to have you cut their hair. This, unfortunately, explains why many barbers are asked to leave the barbering booths for more efficient barbers and they'd start thinking that the shop owner is getting back at them for a flimsy reason.

Know Your Job Specification as a Barber:-it's responsibility as a barber to schedule an appointment with clients where necessary. You also find out from them regularly, how they feel about the hairstyle or shave that you're given, to know if there's a need for improvement.

Apart from cutting and shaving hairs, you should interact with your customers to be sure of what you're doing. Since you're expected to be Knowledgeable on aftershave care and related skin services, you're likely to be advising and giving useful information on how, where, and when to apply hair related treatments.

You must as a culture ensure that your equipment is clean and ready before using it on any customer, etc.

Take Care of Your Physical Appearance:-you should not dress like a Californian gangster; just as having an appearance of a top accounting manager may not be necessary. A very popular adage has it that your dressing tells a lot of story about you.

Although in barbershop business, there's no known dress code; that should not make you casual with your appearance; especially if you're hoping to get employed in a classic barbershop that has a certain category of persons as customers (high-end middle-class individuals).

Why would you worry about your appearance since the job is relatively a rough and messy kind? You may be asking. Apart from the fact that it enhances your personality, it gives a good impression of your level of decency in society.

Personally, Market Yourself:-you can promote yourself in many ways; Social media would make you popular as a barber, but this kind of popularity will depend on the number of positive reviews on your page. Not until you're sure of a large chunk of positive appraisal of your Barbershop services, you should stay away from social media. Keep in mind also, the fact that other barbers are not your enemy; rather are just like you, trying to have a fair market share of the industry.

Hence, when you beat the competition, your barbershop will excel. In no way should you talk bad about others; if you must talk about other barbers, be objective while marketing yourself. For instance, a customer who complains of having his hair spoiled by a certain barber should be advised not to entirely lose hope in the said barber.

Yes! This works like magic; it makes you appear selfless in the eye of the customer and would work in your favor sometime in the future: if you happen to make a mistake while cutting the same person's hair.

Again, your customers will see you as a good person who does not talk down on others; believe it or not, this has a way of keeping them emotionally connected to you. The main issue here is that you should not portray yourself as the best, just allow your customers to do the judgment.

Signpost:- like every other kind of business, you need a sign that should get the attention of passersby. It may be a sign with directional arrows, a bold brand name sign, open for business signs, etc. Banners and Billboardsalso come in handy in this area. Don't also forget to always indicate when the shop is not in operation. It shows courtesy and enhances professionalism.

In planning for your signpost, do remember to add Barbershop-related images that would idealistically say the word Barbershop, even without the word written on it as most persons would notice that more easily than a conventional signpost of who we are and what we do inscription.

CHAPTER 4

Ethical Issues for Barbers

YES, like every other profession, the Barber and the barbering profession are governed by certain moral obligations, which anyone hoping to succeed in the business, should see as a guide.

This moral burden as some have described it often goes unnoticed, but subtly plays an important part, in the sub-consciousness of barbershop customers.

It's a known fact that integrity is in the core, of the need to adhere to an ethics of a given profession; this is because integrity per se, helps one immensely, in managing customer relations; and as such, you should learn to conduct yourself honestly, in your daily transaction with each person.

It's your level of personal integrity that helps you in ensuring that every customer is treated as important as others, despite their financial position in society, or the extra pay you do receive from them.

It's just normal for you to wish for special attention to that customer who gives you extra pay each time you handle his or her hair, the only concern with this is when you allow such an urge to interfere with the way you attend to a second customer who may have entered your barbershop simultaneously with your special customer or even before the fellow.

Though most of those who normally pay a little extra above the normal price to Barbers,

49

after a haircut, is not necessarily asking for special attention; as I have observed in my many years on the job. It's just a way of life for these persons.

We can't also throw away the fact that some would do this as a way of suggesting that they're more important than others, and as such should be given special attention, anytime they come around.

Such preferential treatment, however, should be done in moderation and in fairness to others who might not necessarily give you extra money but are surely among your loyal customers.

In essence, every customer should be attended to, according to how they came. You must not be seen to be favoring a particular person, in such a way as to make another customer feel less important. If you do such a thing, then you'll not only be losing your customers gradually but would be violating the ethics of the profession.

Another way you can ensure that your Barbershop continues to attract the right customers that will sustain its profitability is to have respect for your customers, as an individual and as a customer, whose opinion, you must listen to.

Respecting the feelings, likes, dislikes, and suggestions of your customers, in particular, is a fast way of attracting loyal customers.

Operating a barbershop is very tasking, and sometimes boring, I must say; because you're expected to open for business early and close late. But whether you close early or open late, it all depends on your fitness level and availability.

The most important fact to note is that you must be consistent and your customers will naturally flow along with you. This is where responsibility comes to play. Inconsistency in this area is a bad way of running the business and does not portray you as one who is ethically responsible.

Remember also to always recognize your customers in their persons rather than as a group. If you're already handling clients in a Barbershop, you'll understand better what this aspect of self-recognition is all about.

The truth is that barbershop customers hate telling their barber of their hairstyle always. They expect you to know the regular style since they come to your shop always. And so are angry often if they had to describe the hairstyle each time they come.

By now you're already aware that a lot of conversations take place in the Barbershop. Gossips and some other serious and personal discussions with customers should be kept secret; either in the course of rendering services to them or any other time. I repeat; it should be kept secret.

If it must be mentioned among other customers, reference should not be made of the source, by so doing, you're ensuring the confidentiality of your customers.

Barbers must accept responsibility for their actions and are accountable when necessary if your customer's satisfaction is anything to go by.

CHAPTER 5

Clipper Maintenance And Blade Sharpening

It's one thing to know how to use a hair clipper, to cut and design a hairstyle, but it's entirely a different thing, to know how to do a minor repair on it; for efficiency and effectiveness.

Very few Barbers know these maintenance tips, and that is why many inexperienced Barbers are sometimes seen struggling with their clippers while cutting customer's hair.

What an embarrassing way of letting your customer know that your Barbing knowledge is limited!

If you're a Barber, or that you're familiar with how a hair clipper work, you will agree with me that at one time or the other, you may have come across a troublesome clipper that simply refuses to cut hair the normal way, even after trying all the clipper setting and alignment tricks you'd learn as a Barber.

Perhaps while learning how to be a Barber, you were enthusiastically engrossed about the prospect of becoming a good hair expert that you fail to give attention to this area of Barbing activity that could make or mare your skill.

Without mincing words here, I would say categorically that I had a similar experience, back then as a beginner barber. I had to struggle with it until I open my own Barbershop.

That is, after many years of doing what I hate to do as a sole barber in a Barbershop: I'll use a clipper for a week or so and spend about four hours later in a blade sharpening outlet.

Apart from the fact that I had to lose customers who need a haircut while I was out to sharpen my blade, I often get disappointed when the blade would still not cut fine, after much wasted time. The key to avoiding this is simply learning how to do it yourself.

Ignore the fact that some Clipper blades do not need sharpening: only require cleaning. The reason is that my research has shown that most professional Barbers will always have a need to sharpen blades, as almost all the professional clipper blades that I've used, will work again and even better after it must have undergone a sharpening process.

Hence, honing your professional Clipper blade will save you from the ensuing issue of ragged, hold up, and irregular cuts.

Two months after I opened my first barbershop, I ran into a guy named Kinsley. I knew him two years back, while he was working in a Blade sharpening store, back then in my neighborhood.

Kinsley told me that he was looking for a barbing job because his workplace went under when state authority demolished his makeshift structure that he was using to make a livelihood; after which he could not raise funds to rent a conventional shop to continue his business.

I quickly employed him as one of my Barbers, not because I needed more barbers, but because I was hoping to learn the blade honing skills. Sooner, we worked together. The skills I learn from Kingsley opened a new chapter in my Barbershop business.

So I will share with you how you can conveniently sharpen your clipper blade regularly as soon as the cutting edge gets dull.

All you need is:

1. A **sharpening stone** or **whetstone**:- Note that you need an oil stone of certain grit, perhaps 4000 grit up to 8000 grit for smoother finishing; unless you're having a ceramic blade, then you will require a diamond Sharpening stone.

   A Clean Towel:- a piece of cloths or similar material, to be used for cleaning dirt.

   A cleaning Agent:-**Isopropyl** alcohol is preferable. It helps to clean invisible dirty, including rust, and leaves the Blade shiny and clean; so that the blade would sharpen properly

   A Clean Hair Brush:-for removing the heavy debris and corrosion that might have built up within the blades

2. **A Small Bowl:** for alcohol blade-washing; and a **Clipper oil**

   Unless you're sure that the blade is due for sharpening, do not sharpen. Perhaps, just by disassembling the blades, wiping off dirt, cleaning with at least 90% alcohol, and reassembling, may get it back to service.

As a Barber, I believe you already know how to lose and tighten your clipper blade, in a proper manner. If you cannot conveniently pair Clipper blades in the right way, then you need to go back to your Barber school, because it's what you will be doing on a regular interval. Improperly aligned Clipper blade will not cut hair correctly, and I guess you don't want to be seen fumbling in front of your customers.

Now sharpening the blades:- By now you must have removed the usual two screws on either side of the bigger blade; you've rinsed it with a cleaning agent, as discussed above; use the clean towel to wipe the blade dry and ready to be honed.

If you're using an oil stone, apply a little drop of clipper oil on the surface of the stone (4000 grit surface) and evenly distribute it.

You can use almost anything that can hold the blade in place while you rub the inner surface of the blade on the stone. Some recommend using a strong magnet that can trap the blade firmly. If you can't find anything that can hold the blade, use adhesive tape, rolled and attached to the back of the blade; then place your hand on it and rub gently up and down, (not recommended because of hurting your hand if it gets very hot) till the blade becomes hot. You will change the position of the blade regularly and continue honing it until you're satisfied.

Use the smoother surface stone (8000 grit surface) to complete the process.
The glittering surface of the blade will tell you when it's well sharpened. With experience also, you will notice the sharpness by feeling the edge with the tip of your finger; but a good indicator is the very-clean-brightness of its surface and a certain degree of hotness of the blade.

Note that your hand may get messy with particles of the stone and the oil. Do not worry it's a manual process you can adopt for an emergency unless you have the horning machine or you decide to have many spear blades to switch to, while the dull ones are sent to those who do the sharpening services.

When you're through with the first blade, you repeat the process on the second blade.

After this process, you fix the blade on the Clipper and apply Clipper oil before turning on the machine. Allow it to run for about two minutes or so to allow it to be friction-ready/free.   Then you're ready to continue your barbing with a sharper edge blade.

CHAPTER 6

Things That Gives Professional Barbers Money

The haircutting industry is a creative–laden industry. And like all other creative professions, your success rate is dependent on your personal ability to creatively establish your skill in the industry rather than the knowledge acquired as a Barber.

So those who found themselves in the profession, regardless of their level of education, are capable of achieving almost anything achievable. That is why I have compiled below the possible ways in which a 21st-century barber can make money. The only thing needed of you is to be perfect on the job with good reviews from your customers, daily.

Opening a Barbershop: - One major way you can make your own money as a barber is by establishing your own Barbershop. By doing this you have become a business owner; and with the right application of entrepreneurial knowledge in the business, the sky should be your limit.

While rendering barbering services to your clients, you can employ other barbers, if your customer base is way above your capability or if there's a need for expansion.

Hiring a Suite:-assuming you don't have enough finance to establish a barbershop, you may go into a business deal with an already existing business organization like Hotels, leisure centers, and business Malls, etc. where you use a section of the company's building to operate your barbershop. Income generated is usually shared between you and the management, depending on the arrangement. Some business organizations may require remission of a certain amount of money daily, weekly, or monthly as the case may be. Others would rent the space for you and you make a payment on an installment basis.

Booth Rental:- most standard Barbershops are designed in such a way as to have many barber's chairs and its mirror; each Barber's chair or booth is occupied by a barber. Most barbers who work in those booths are placed either on salary, commission, or booth rental.

With this, the Barber is expected to pay a certain amount of money daily or weekly, depending on the arrangement with the owner of the Business. So as a barber, if you don't have money to open a shop, you can rent a booth and make your money.

Work from home Barbers:-You can start your Barbershop from your living apartment. In this case, you furnish a section of a room for this purpose, with a good signpost at a strategic location, you render barbering services.

The home-based barber makes more money if they have an established customer base already within the locality, as they would not only connect personally with individual customers who believe in their skill but will be more free and ready to go for Home-services on high ranking individuals who often invite barbers to their private home for their haircut, rather than using a Barbershop.

Barbers with many of these wealthy kinds of customers will make more money as most of these individuals pay a very high amount for Home-Services.

Working on commission:- as a Barber, you can take up a job in a Barbershop with a reasonable number of customers, where you work on a commission that would be determined by the owner of the shop.

Most freelance Barbers embrace this method, as their commitment level to the growth of the business are usually very low; only interested in the number of customers they can attend to. The more the number, the higher their payment, as the percentage of an amount realized is given to them.

In my locality, it's usually $30 for every $90 earned. Barbershop owners will not employ you for commission if they're not sure of your expertise.

Mobile Barber:- the rate at which technology is advancing has necessitated a mobile Barber arrangement. With the numerous advantages of social media advertising, a Barber can set up a virtual online shop for a purpose of connecting with prospective customers, after which an appointment is scheduled for the Barber, who takes his services to the doorstep of the client.

Booking can be done online, through telephone, or face-to-face. This will appeal to a client who requires some kind of privacy always; like celebrities and those who hate to stay behind waiting for their turn in a

Barbershop. The appointment is usually scheduled based on the convenience and availability of both the Barber and the client that booked the Barber.

Operating a Barber School:- this is an area that required very little compared to what many would be thinking. An average Barbershop is capable of running a Barber school.

Having fulfilled the local licensing requirement for this, you can turn a section of that your barbershop into a school for grooming of young lads who are interested in learning the job.

You'll be amazed at the number of persons who will be willing to enroll, and the income that would accrue thereof; provided that inexperience barbers are not allowed to interface with real customers of the Barbershop to avoid a wrong impression that could arise when the client who complains of spoiled hairstyle would learn that an amateur did the job on him or her.

Consultancy and Product Marketing:- As a professional barber, people would consult you daily to ask questions about men's beauty, the right hair care products minor clipper fixing, and related services.

Barbers do not only make money from referring and selling these products to clients but would charge fees for minor services that would include but not limited to acting as a middle man between the seller and the buyer of certain Barbershop related products and services.

Public Speaking and Sponsorship:- who says you cannot become famous as a Berber when you can be called upon to deliver a barbering lecture to Learners, as a veteran Barber. If your barbershop brand is very famous it can also attract partnerships or even sponsorship from manufacturers of barbershop products.

CHAPTER 7

What You Need To Know Before Establishing A Barbershop

Before you abandon that your regular 9 to 5 job for a Barbershop business it would be okay if you make out time to understand a few things that obviously would determine your success rate in the business. For this write-up, I will say here that unless you work and earn a daily income in a Barbershop, you're not supposed to be called a Barber.

This presupposes that knowing how to cut men's hair or having a certificate from a barber school is not a guarantee that you're ready to excel in the barbering business. That's why you need to consider certain things about a Barber that makes them succeed or fail in the business.

As a seasoned Barber with many years' experience, I'll tell you a few realities that are unique in the life of professional Barbers and Barbershop owners. That, unfortunately, constitutes the downside of the job.

Work-life Balance and schedules:- you must not go into the Barbering business just because you think that some guys down the street are making a lot of cash in it; or that the demand is quite high in your neighborhood, so you want to cash in on it.

The working pattern of an average Barber is so unique that you have to work more when others are resting and holidaying. That's why you have to be prepared to sacrifice a lot about your social life. As you already know,

Barbers are usually very busy during festive holidays like Christmas; and other public holidays.

Even though you're expected to open for service, as early as possible, you will likely be closing the shop late; because when the regular 9 to 5 workers are returning from work, that's when a larger portion of your customers would be coming in to have their hairs worked on.

The same is the case with weekends that you have to grapple with the influx of customers. What this means is that you would most likely be missing out on those special social functions that are usually held on weekends and public holidays; simply because you're tied down with fellows who want to look good for the same occasion.

 What if my Barbershop runs a shift schedule and I decide to take off duty? You may be asking; sure, you can decide whether to work or not on these special periods, but that's definitely against the norm.

Your absence within this special period that your customers want you most, to improve their appearance is a way of telling them that you're not serious in the business. It's worse if you're the only one working in the shop, as the shop would remain shut until you resume service. As a married fellow in this unique Barbershop schedule, be assured that your partner will always feel lonely if you have to spend more of these special periods working.

I will say this without any reservation that a lot of successful professional Barbers are having it tough with their significant order because of this constant-work lifestyle. No wonder the majority of those who initially were enthusiastic about Barber's lifestyle is likely to abandon the job within three years.

Very few who would continue, are only held because of the financial benefit that they're getting at the moment, not because they hope to progress in the career.

Being a Licensed Barber:- as I've already noted, graduating from a Barber school is just the first step that you have to take. You need to be passionate about the job. It's rather funny how folks fizzle out of the job for some flimsy reasons. The very many that I have spoken to on this, after spending money to acquire the Barbering skill did agree that they found out in practice, that the passion for the job isn't there.

I concluded that it's either because of the real nature of the job or their lack of creative ingenuity that is required for the job.

No wonder many would rather transitions to other jobs at the slightest opportunity but not knowing exactly why they have to. And as you would soon find out, when passion is lacking in this kind of job stress and exhaustion is usually the case.

Barbering is energy-draining:- like all jobs that are done manually, a barber should be physically ready to adapt to the fitness level required. Apart from the long hours that you have to stand to churn out a perfect haircut, the effect of constant arm movement and stretching of the upper limb joints is something you need to consider.

This constant angling and craning that Barbers go through involve lots of mental processes too. To say the obvious, you need to be healthy and physically fit for the job.

Are you a qualified Barber?:- let me remind you once again that running a Barbershop is far above just being certified as a graduate Barber, from a reputable Barber's school; otherwise, you'd discover soon that customers know those that are expert Barbers and those who are yet to perfect on the skills.

Even those that do not know how the Hair Clipper works can tell who's a learner from the pros, simply by the way the clipper is clipping their hair.

The best way to overcome this odd is to try having internship experience with an expert Barber who will help you grow in practical skill and confidence.

Most barbershops would accept your offer to do an internship if there's no monetary reward attached. In such a situation you'd be confined to less tasking Hairstyles; especially that of minors that would not pose many challenges to you, until you're ready for a bigger task.

Though you might want to try a bigger task while doing this, always seek the "senior" Barber's approval to avoid creating the wrong impression that would affect his business.

You can move from internship to percentage earning barber, as most Barbershop owners would also be willing to place you on their payroll as soon as they discover that customers are attesting to your skill.

This, apart from helping you to perfect, would expose you to other routine tasks that hitherto was not known to you; and such things are never taught in the school, only obvious when you start attending to customers in a barbershop.

Legal issue and licensing:- remember to adhere to local laws regarding the establishment of a Barbershop and licensing of Barbers. I also know that in some regions, barbers still operate in their primitive pattern, where anyone can just rent a shop and start attending to customers who do not also care about the legality of such a shop.

This is usually the case in my home country where the majority of the barbers do not even have a formal Barber education and are not eager to acquire any. Most got their Barbering skill through internship and one-on-one tutoring that are not comprehensive when compared to what is been taught in an organized Barber school.

Modern states like the US and many parts of Europe are ensuring that Barbers are licensed appropriately like other professions.

Remember The Social Aspect Of The Job:- yes! The job of a Barber is such that goes hand-in-hand with meeting different people every day and constantly interacting interpersonally with them. If you're the type that is blessed with a likable personality, it's a plus to your skill, as most guys would want to identify with your shop because of your relationship with them.

I still remember the kind of bond that I felt then with my Barbershop customers when I had to regrettably apologize for not being able to handle their hair when they need it arranged. The bonding is even more thrilling if they had to stay that way (without cutting their hair) until you return from where ever you must have been.

It's this passionate aspect of the job that would define whether you would succeed in building a community of followers that would keep your barbershop running for a long time.

The unlicensed Barber:- As an entrepreneur, you're interested in investing in the Barbershop business? Perhaps, you have a special interest in the cosmetic industry, especially the Barbering sector. I also assume you have gone through an internship informally, hence are yet to be certified.

You too can succeed in this industry, provided that you follow the required process and understand the necessaries of running a Barbershop. Apart from reading books like this and applying what you already know as an entrepreneur, you can employ a licensed barber to begin the process; while you fortified yourself to take over as soon as possible.

Though very few materials are available for study online about Barbering, you need to search and study Barbering rules, Anatomy and physiology, health and safety on hazardous subjects like HIV/AIDS and related disease control, disinfection and sanitation, as well as hair care and treatment; because these subjects are central to what is been taught in most Barber school.

Other aspects of the job like Haircutting, Shaving, Permanent Waving, Hair Relaxing,

Hair Coloring, Shampooing, etc. are better understood when you do them practically

CHAPTER 8

Basic Barbershop Tools

The following tools or equipment is what you need in your Barbershop, though you may not use some of them as often as you use others but still, you need to make sure that they're available on demand.

The Hair Clipper:- investing in a good brand of clipper for your barbershop is always a plus for the business. Whether it's a direct current electric clipper, rechargeable or replaceable-battery clipper, all that's required is a clipper that can carry out the hair cutting task perfectly.

As a rule, it's always better to have a spear clipper for each Barber's booth, to avoid circumstantial delays that are normal though.

This is because no matter how good a clipper might be, certain hair conditions can make them malfunction suddenly.

These conditions include very oily hairs with a lot of debris that can allow unnecessary dirt into the blade cutting edge, which would make it less effective in clipping hairs.

Another could be an excessively used blade that requires sharpening, which could suddenly malfunctions especially when such a blade is used on a very tough hair. Again the adjustable setting of the clipper blade could shift from its normal position while in use.

In each of these scenarios, trying to fix the clipper while the customer is waiting is usually not the best; rather you're expected to immediately switch to a standby clipper.

81

Based on the foregoing, you will need as many clippers as possible depending on the size of your shop or the number of barber's booths available.

Chairs: - there are specific types of chairs best suited for this job. They're the adjustable swivels chairs. With this chair, you can adjust up and down the height of the chair to suit your best barbering position.

This swivel chair also allows 360 degrees turning of your subject, which makes your work easier while facing the mirror.

HairComb/Brush:- you will need a set of comb with different shapes and sizes, for various levels of hairs and hairstyles; as well as a hairbrush.

Scissors:- the scissors would be useful for a certain kind of cutting and trimming. Though creative barbers can use the clipper to achieve almost everything the scissors would do on a hair.

Mirror:- the mirror does not need any explanation here as both the Barber and his customer would regularly use the mirror throughout the hair cutting period.

Straight Razor/ Smooth Shaver:- the straight razor is used to clean hairs on a certain area of the head, especially around the neck region, to make a smooth shave.

It's a traditional Barbershop tool that has also been modified by technology, as most barbers now have the option of using many brands of electric smooth shavers that can achieve similar results with the traditional razor. Anyone you decide to use should be based on your skill and customers' need.

Cape:- is the name used in describing that covering material that is usually used in shielding customers body from dropping hairs. The cape is designed to prevent hairs from settling on people's cloth or skin while having a haircut. The barber can as well have one for himself designed for the same purpose, depending on his choice.

Nose Trimmer:- it's a little device that is usually powered by an AA sized battery, used to remove hairs from the nose and ear region. It makes the barbershop look professional and appealing to men, especially older males who request mostly this kind of nose service.

Disinfectant and Sterilizers:- you will need a good disinfectant like isopropyl alcohol, for regular cleaning of your equipment. And when necessary, tools like clippers, shavers, scissors, and similar blades are kept in sterile conditions in a sterilizing machine specially designed for Barbershops and related services.

Hair Care and Shaving Products:-good brand of creams, oil, and related lotions should be available in your shop, to help in softening and conditioning of hairs, and for achieving a smooth shave; as well as in treating hair related skin infections like dandruff and the likes.

Hair Dryer:- you might also need a hairdryer, especially the handheld ones, in case you have a customer that needs such a blow-dryer service. It's, however, a must for a barber that can also style both male and female hairs.

Towel Warmer:- it would be very useful to invest in a very good brand of towel warming machine, that should take care of those in love with the Hot-towel shave. Most barbershop owners, who know about the benefit of this, use it to gain a competitive edge over their competitors.

Other Equipment:- other things that you would need would depend so much on your Budget and the Barbershop design that you want to adopt.

In any case always remember the inevitable role of using the right furniture for customers waiting for their turn, proper air conditioning system, and a glass cabinet for storing of kits, usually with a transparent glass panel to showcase available products and supplies. Not forgetting, of course, a good wall hanger for Barber props like the cape, etc.

CHAPTER 9

On the job advice for a barber

Perhaps you have rightly set up your barbershop, gotten the required licenses, and are ready to hit the ground running; with the "open for barbershop services" sign already turned on. Congratulation though!

But before you miss an important aspect that may decide your success or failure as the case may be. Earlier, I said something about "no two hairs grow the same way" meaning that every individual's hair has a unique texture and growth pattern that is a function of once race (black or white), region(an American or an Asian), and sometimes country of origin.

 I'm saying this because I was opportune to work in a high-end Barbershop some years back that was located near a border post.

Though 80% of the customers were generally black Africans, once or twice a day, I find myself cutting a foreigner with somewhat fragile long hairs.

This is where your professionalism is required the most, so you don't turn a customer's medium-length hairstyle into a short-length, simply because you do not understand the nature of the hair (the natural curl of the soft or hard texture of the hair).

As a barber, medium-length hairstyles like the faux hawks and the pompadours are among the easiest male styles for those with long hairs but it's often, a nightmare for armature barbers.

The truth is that every professional Barber should know how those hair follicles grow and develop a special skill to handle the numerous variations of the medium and short-length hairstyles

In my location, based on contemporary trend; most of the male customers would want it short on the sides, and a perfect cut on the top that might be as high as between 5 and 10cm. so all I did was to perfect my skill very well in that area.

As such, even if I have a rush, I will simply stick to an imaginary template in my brain to give everyone a perfect cut.

You don't want to be caught up in a usual scenario that worries armature barbers: you're working on a hair without an idea of how the final shape will be; you're just hoping that the hairstyle will somehow take an accidental shape.

Know also that apart from those that already have a permanent style, a lot of people will want you to choose a style for them, and naturally, you may want to choose an easier style. I'd rather suggest you choose a trendy style if you think that the fellow is somewhat trendy based on appearance, or just give a perfect hairstyle that suits the natural pattern of the head and hair growth; to enhance the beauty of the face.

CHAPTER 10

Operational Skills That Can Help A Barber To Succeed

Because of the high increase in the number of people requiring a nice haircut and the attendant attention to hair and beard styling, especially in today's men fashion, any barber or barbershop that want to remain relevant must know what to do.

If you want to constantly make a good impression that will keep your customers coming back to you, you must not only have proper barbering training, which is in high demand, you must be familiar with the traditional barber cut, trim, and styling of shorter hair.

Your focus may be on the men, because you're running a strictly-for men's barbershop, as against a unisex beauty shop; remember that women with shorter hair are more comfortable with a barber for their styling.

Contemporary male fashion is fast changing; this also includes barbering skills. Modern barbers are improving in their knowledge of the various facial and hair service creativity.

Most people now require a unique custom look that very skillful barbers should achieve through creative shaping and styling

Apart from enrolling in an atypical Barber Program and learning the basic barbering skill, you need to read and learn more about the barber as a career.

I assume you have acquired the basic qualifications. I also assume that you have been cutting hairs for folks who often drop good reviews about the high level of your creativity.

As funny as this may sound, it's also possible that you are not interested in how you can become a career Barber. You're just satisfied cutting hairs and getting the compliments and hoping to take up a better job in a more lucrative industry.

If my guess is wrong, perhaps you're interested in being a household name in the hair grooming and styling industry, you have indeed picked the right lesson that should teach you more things that you never thought were important.

Doing the hair cutting

One of the first things that I have always told learner barbers is the fact that hair types differ from person to person. And it's not enough to know this but understanding and developing a unique technique that should enable you to handle these variants of hair growth pattern

If you understand this then you're better equipped to follow the ever-changing trend in men's beauty and grooming.

Contemporary men's haircut requires special barbering skills and staying up to date on the newest hairstyles; especially if your aim is not just to cut hairs and have people tell you thanks, but to grow your barbershop into a model to be followed by others.

Having acquired the requisite cosmetology license that should give your barbershop a go-ahead order, and your skills are good enough to set and maintain a barbering standard, it's just one more thing that I have to say before you go: listen very carefully to your customers.

Listening skill

Almost all the category of work done in the hair beauty and cosmetology industry requires you to become talented at listening and interpreting client's requests.

Hair Trimming

This is one major area that is often overlooked or done with a carefree attitude, by most barbers who often become overconfident about their ability.

This is bad because the customers that will make your business stay afloat are your loyal customers, and most of your loyal customers in this profession are those you have given a good hair design to their hairs, they liked it and thereafter became a regular caller to your barbershop.

These categories of persons often require just light trimming to the hairs because you already know the template of their hairstyle. As a human, you might not be perfect at all the time, but ensure you limit the rate of the error to the barest minimum.

When necessary, try turning a possible mistake into a new unique style; that is what creativity in this profession is all about.

Hair trimming in this regard is what many will call hair maintenance. We all like beauty but some people are more beauty conscious than others. So, once you have created for a client the style that they prefer, they'll want to keep returning to your barbershop for maintenance or trimming.

By this, I'm saying that you should learn how to maintain a hairstyle. Each time you do this trimming, the client will want to see the exact style that he saw initially that made him or her decides to stick to that style, and nothing less. That is why trimming is very tricky and requires more attention than you may think.

Doing this more regularly to most of your customers will not only help increase the number of repeat clients for your barbershop, but it will also give your skill more referrals from happy clients.

Styling

Styling is what you should know as a barbershop operator, if possible specify the styles you can do perfectly but is not necessary because clients just want you to replicate on them any hairstyle that they think will make them trendy. Some will want it just the way they see it on certain personalities, like celebrities, or even what they see on TV, online, and in periodicals.

Though you might not learn all the styles at once because styles themselves are dynamic: changing with time and trend, but the basic styling techniques for barbers that you learned in your cosmetology school is enough to take care of every style.

I also know that some specific programs that focus on men's styling, will equip you more with advanced skills that should help you to take care of traditional and fashionable hairstyling scheme.

Shaping

A sharp and straight line is the keyword for shaping; it's not just enough to shape a hair, your shaping should not show an irregular line or a shaky line. I hope you still remember your lesson on clipper handling: how you hold the clipper why shaping a hair has a lot to tell of the possible outcome of the shaping.

You must master this skillful art on the beard region; as well as the hairlines of your clients. People with shorter haircuts require more clean shaping; that clean shaping that brings out the perfect cut you see people admire.

You will not know what this line means to some persons until you mess up their hair or beard lines. So as a professional barber, you must ensure clean lines and be precise in shaping.

Shaving

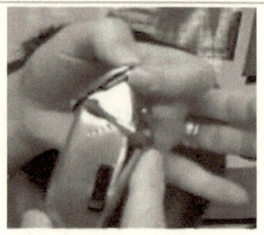

Do you still remember the shaving techniques you learned, while preparing yourself for this beauty profession- do you still remember that Straight razor shaving is very key to your licensing as a barber? Assuming you have forgotten, let me re-echo the importance of this to you because it's as old as the barbering profession.

As they say, a smooth straight Razor shave remains one of the qualities of a good barber. Almost everyone enjoys that clean feel of a very close shave and as such, professionals barbers that do this perfectly as part of their services, are an edge over those who do not.

Though it takes some training and practice to perfect on this job; developing specific skills and being dedicated to the art of men's styling, is a major need to achieving success.

Don't also forget that you need to have a good knowledge of skincare because some persons would need advice on that area more often.

Make your Services Regular and consistent

Always open your barbershop on time as you have advertised. Remember the last-minute customer, he or she deserves to be attended to.

Occasionally you may turn down a request to stay a little behind schedule by this category of customers; it should however be done with a good reason that should be well explained to the customer.

Now, while attending to that late-comer customer, don't always expect a kind of kick-back, in form of extra money as most will promise, just to make you agree to render the service to them.

It should be done strictly base on the perceived need of the customer. Notwithstanding, you will always receive a good tip or even win loyal customers in this way.

It's really difficult to ascertain how customers feel about your skill or what they'd miss without you until you put yourself in their shoes and be appreciative of what they experience around you.

CHAPTER 11

Haircut Numbers or Hair Clipper Sizes

One of the things you would not want to happen is to allow your customers to tell you what you're supposed to know as a Barber. One of such things is to know the various levels of hairs or the sizes of the clipper, as the case may be.

I imagine someone entering your barbing booth and simply telling you to give him or her a cut. The next question from you naturally will be: which of the styles; what type of cut, or how do you want it done, etc.

But if the customer had said: I want a zero cut. This is self-explanatory, as every professional barber should know what a zero cut is. Now this leads us to the main discussion

The question of how long or how short a hair should be has been taken care of by those who designed the hair clipper; through the serial numbering of the sizes. You can achieve these sizes from manipulating the clipper adjustable levers to using the clipper blade guards

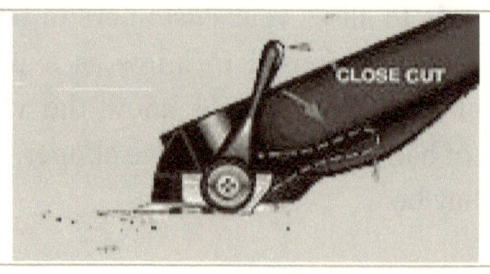

Image of clipper adjustable lever in a close blade position

This numbering can be confusing to a lot of learner barbers, simply because most, do not understand the apparent differences between the hair levels

It's something you need not be confused about, as this is something you will be applying every minute of each haircutting section. Customers may not know exactly the number of inches they want to be removed from their hairs, that's why you hear them say often: "Oh that's too low" or "I think it's still high, I want it down more"

This sometimes confuses especially if the barber doesn't know more about this clipper numbering or sizes. I will be explaining in detail the numbers and what they're meant to do on your hairs.

A clipper number is a clipper haircut guard, usually in different sizes fractionalized between 1, 2, 3, up to 8 guards; as observed in most of the professional clippers.

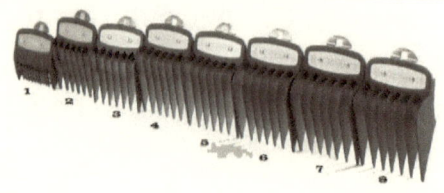

These sizes each represent the quantity of hair that will be left behind if used on a particular hair.

Majorly, what happens is that the bigger the number the longer the hair that will be left behind. Meaning that using a number 5 for instance, will leave more hair on a customer compared to the number 3 size, vice versa.

If I want to give a number 4 cut to a customer for example, and as expected, I already have the mathematical calculation offhand; I'm expecting to leave a hair that is a half of an inch: the 4 divided by 8, calculated mathematically (4/8) or (1/2) of an inch

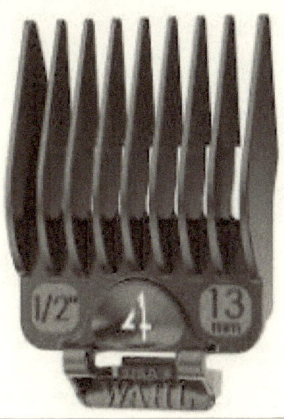

Image of a number 4 clipper guard

But if I decide to give my customer a number 2 cut, my customer will be leaving with a haircut that is one-fourth of an inch: 2 divided by 8 (2/8) or (1/4). As expected, these second cut will be shorter.

There's also a number zero (0) cut, that is achieved when you want to create a near-smooth skin shave. The zero cut will not require a guard.

Base on what I have stated above, using any of the numbers will give you results as follows:

1st clipper size will leave hair that is one-eighth of an inch

2nd clipper size will leave hair that is two-eights of an inch, otherwise referred to as one-quarter of an inch

3rd clipper size leaves three-eighths of an inch

While the 4th clipper size will leave half of an inch

Similarly, the 5th size leaves five-eighths of an inch, 6th size leaves six-eights, better known as three- quarters of an inch, 7th size: seven-eighths; while the last number, the 8th size will leave a one-inch hair on the head.

Below is a computer-generated image that represents levels of hairs from a zero cut to the 7th cut

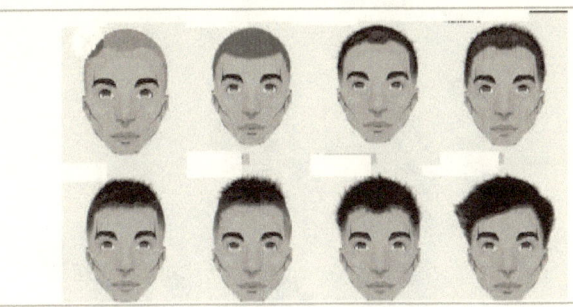

Levels of hairs from zero cut to the 7th cut

ZERO HAIRCUTS

If you want a cut that is very short, close to a razor shave, or just a bald_fade, the clipper guards are not needed here. It's the shortest haircut you can do with the clipper. It exposes the scalp in some way, so if you don't want to reveal the nature of your scalp, always avoid the zero cut

There are lots of variations to the zero cut, depending on the position of the adjustable clipper lever. You can open it and do a Zero cut similar to the image below.

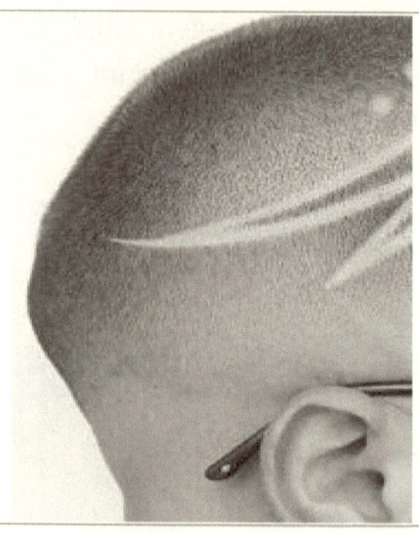

The upper part of the image above is achieved with a zero cut clipper size that has its adjustable lever opened, while the lower part was done with a closed lever. Somewhere in-between the upper and the lower level is achieved through constant manipulation of the adjustable lever to either open or close, close and open, in no particular order.

That is where the creativity of the Barber comes to play. As can be observed in this image

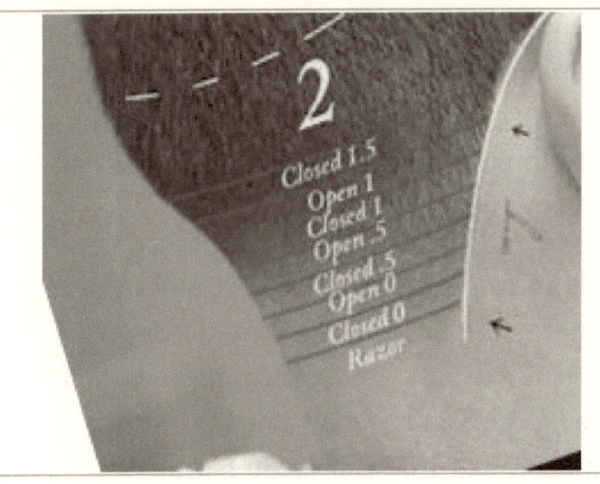

1ST LEVEL HAIRCUT

The number one haircut has more hair than the zero cut. As stated earlier, you can do this cut by attaching the number 1 clipper blade guard.

You will have a haircut that is about *1/8 of an inch*. Let me also state that it's sometimes confusing to decide haircut number, just by looking at the haircut because of the differences in nature and texture of human hairs.

Though experience barbers will always know what to do once they see a sample image of what a customer wants; you can also experiment with one or two levels of the clipper guard.

This is to see which one best suits the style, since a number one haircut on a very thick African hair designed with a number 3 clipper size, for instance, may not appear the same with soft textured European hair.

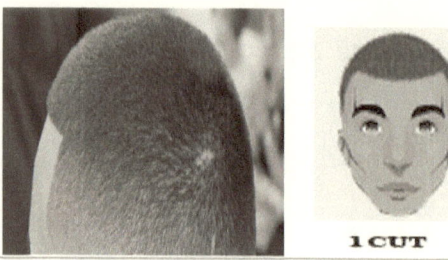

1 CUT

Realistic image of Number 1 cut

2ND LEVEL HAIRCUT

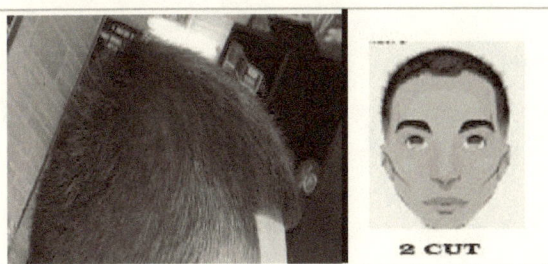

Realistic image of Number 2 cut

' 3RD LEVEL HAIRCUT

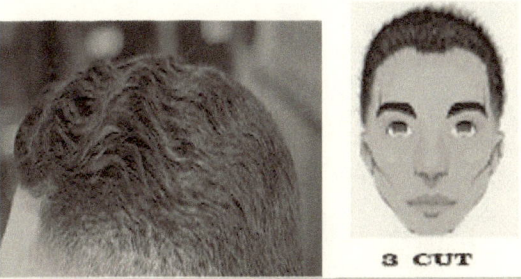

Realistic image of Number 3 cut

www.ingramcontent.com/pod-product-compliance
Lightning Source LLC
Chambersburg PA
CBHW020325290526
45785CB00007B/2921

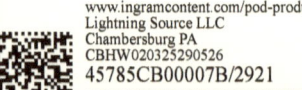